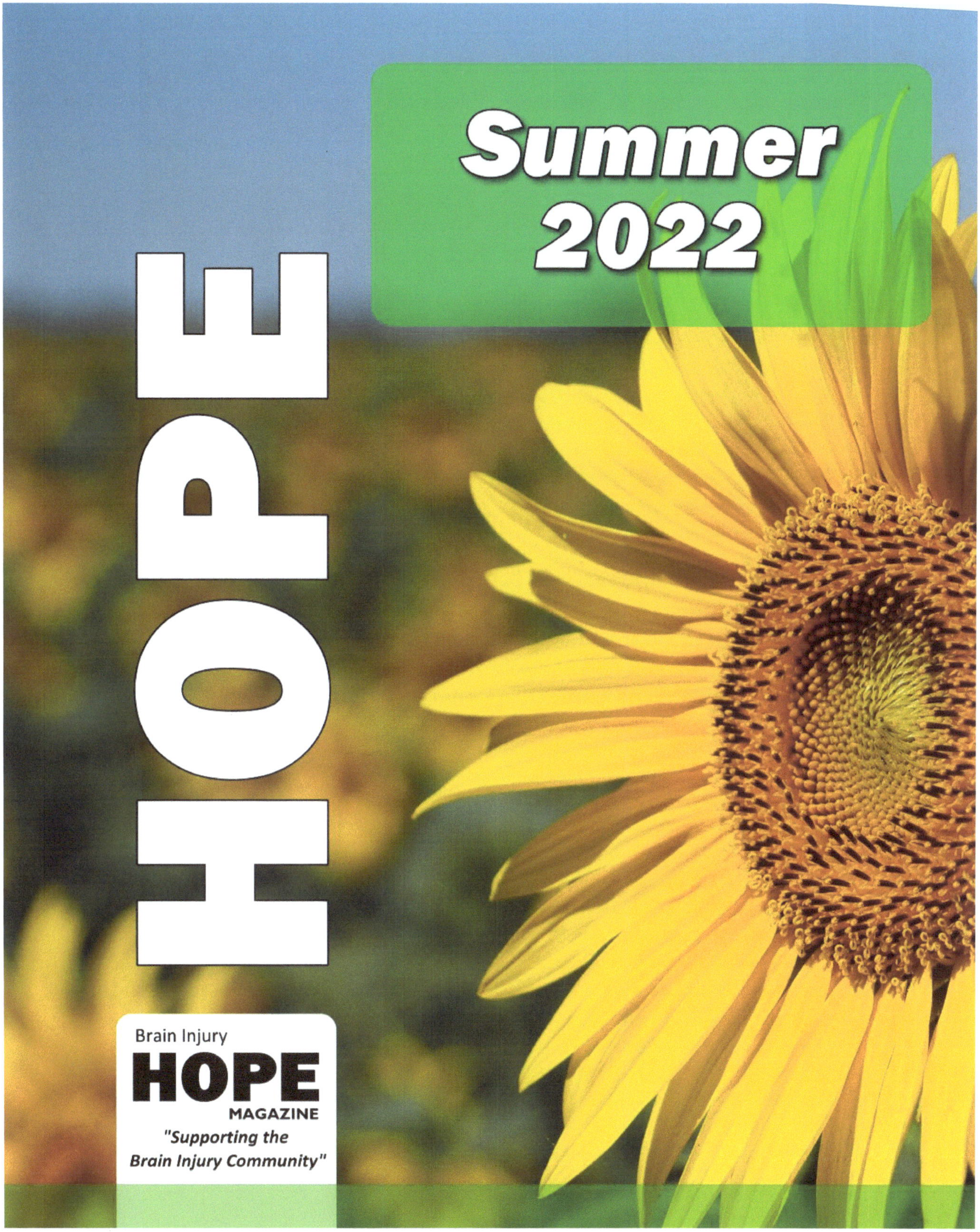

Summer 2022

HOPE

Brain Injury
HOPE
MAGAZINE
*"Supporting the
Brain Injury Community"*

Welcome

HOPE MAGAZINE

Serving the Brain Injury Community

Summer 2022

Publisher
David A. Grant

Editor
Sarah Grant

Our Contributors

Lisa Marie Ansell
Patrick Brigham
Christina Coates
David A. Grant
Natalie McDonald
Isaac Peterson
Scott Smythe

Welcome to the Summer 2022 issue of HOPE Magazine!

When brain injury strikes, especially early on, it's difficult, if not impossible to imagine life ever being good again. Relationships are torn asunder, careers are compromised, finances devasted, and it so often feels like life has been turned completely upside down, that life will never again be worthwhile.

But ask any "brain injury old-timer," and most will tell you that new footing will eventually be found, and that life, albeit different, will become meaningful again.

This issue of HOPE Magazine shares stories of survivors who have found a way to embrace life after brain injury and do so with relative happiness and joy.

I hope you enjoy these stories of true victory of the human spirit.

David A. Grant
Publisher

Table
of Contents

*"Find a place inside where there's joy,
and the joy will burn out the pain."*

-Joseph Campbell

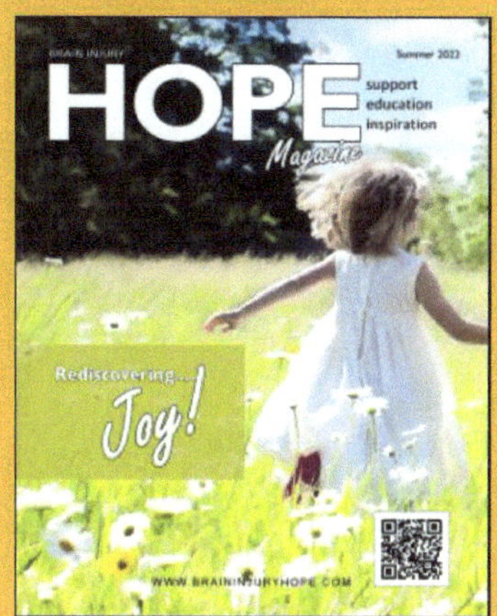

Summer 2022

Advocacy

Education

Inspiration

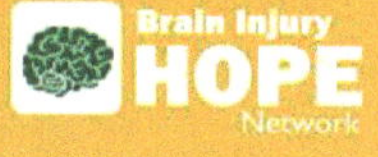

Reflections on my Journey

By Natalie McDonald

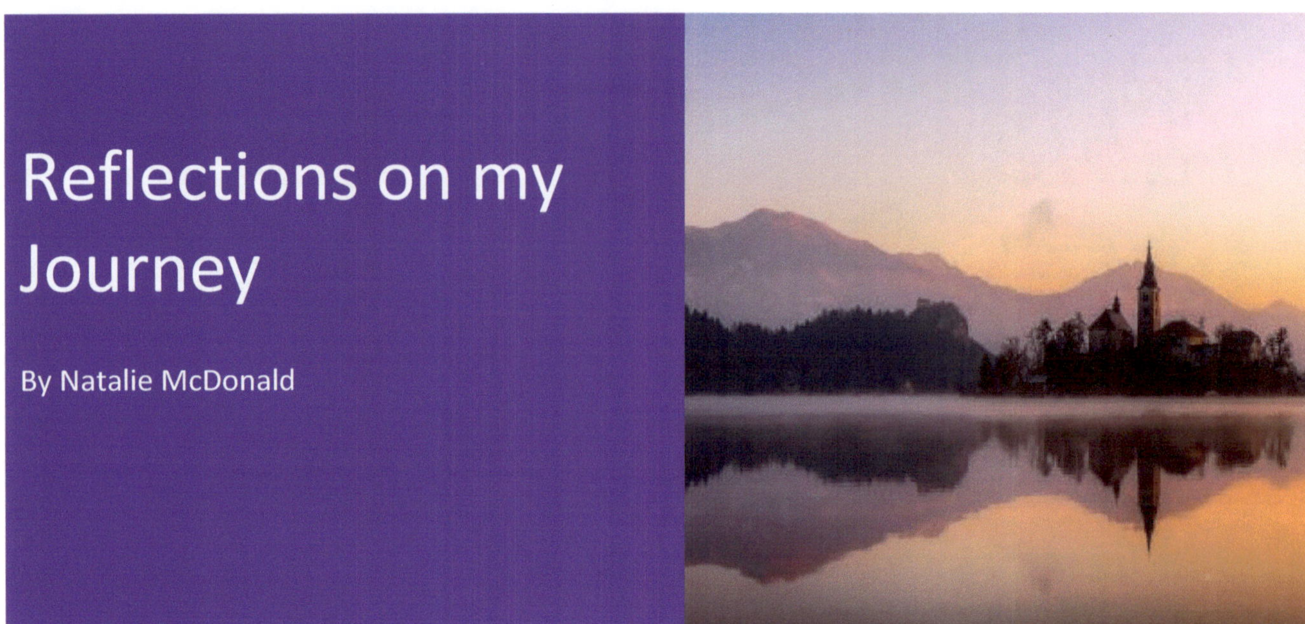

It's been seven and a half years since I began the journey I call "Natalie 2.0." It started one night in September as I drove to my school for an evening musical rehearsal. Back then I was the high school vocal music director at a nearby school district.

As I neared an intersection, a driver in a truck raced through a stop sign and hit my car in the passenger door. People living nearby called 911 and ran to the scene. Finding my phone flung out on the grass, they called my husband and told him the news.

A policewoman arrived at the scene first and climbed in my broken back window to support my neck until emergency crews could get there. She literally saved my life.

> "As I neared an intersection, a driver in a truck raced through a stop sign and hit my car in the passenger door. People living nearby called 911 and ran to the scene."

I almost died of internal bleeding in the ambulance on the way to the hospital. After several surgeries I stayed in the deepest level of coma for about six weeks. Then I started slowly traveling through each level of coma recovery, remaining in some of the more distressing ones for way too long. Eventually I was moved out of ICU to a regular ward. After I began showing signs of consciousness, we finally got insurance approval. I know everyone reading is all too familiar with that concept. I was moved to *On With Life* brain injury rehabilitation facility in Ankeny, IA. I went through months of inpatient therapy and was finally allowed to return home with my husband as my primary caregiver. Our adult daughter and son also took turns living with us for the first two years and drove me to outpatient therapy sessions.

No one could have predicted my journey. For a few years, it seemed that we were just lurching from crisis-to-crisis. Then came the leveling-out years when somber reality started settling in. It seemed to me that there were no more big triumphs, just minor improvements followed by major disappointments.

Although my health had stabilized somewhat, this was a turbulent time for my psyche. I had a strong conviction that since I had survived such a cataclysmic event, something huge should come out of it. I would write a book or become a speaker. Something!

It was necessary to develop some different interests now, things that I hadn't fully pursued because I never had the time. Now I did. And all those years I had "wasted" chasing unrealized goals? They weren't really wasted at all, because without that effort I never would have gotten this far.

These days I have hours to watch birds, squirrels, deer, turkeys, and the occasional groundhog in our yard. I sit and study their behavior. I can take care of our cats, especially our very elderly one (Sirius Black) who is ecstatic at how available I am to now cater to his every need. I'm now midway through my third on-line seminary-level class.

Everything in our lives now is a reason for celebration, starting with the fact that I wake up each morning. Being able to move my legs, feeling my body temperature stabilize (finally), opening my eyes and seeing light flood in, talking, hearing... all these things are miracles for me. I can even make my own meals and cook for our family again.

I write old-fashioned letters to family and friends these days as an "occupational therapy." The act of planning what I'll say, getting it legibly down on the paper, then folding and putting the letter in the envelope (not to mention getting the stamp and return address label in the right place on the envelope!) has been great for me and for my relationships.

> **Everything in our lives now is a reason for celebration, starting with the fact that I wake up each morning.**

I still try to read up on the newest developments in brain plasticity and rehabilitation as well as my own health issues and take any needed actions accordingly. It's not that I have no dreams left. I simply have to be more selective now. It's a good life and we are in peaceful waters these days. I'm not "cured" or even "fixed." We've found there's really never a clear ending to a brain injury journey. But I am healing in very profound ways. I keep discovering new joys, and I know there are more ahead. I have confidence, at least most of the time, that we'll get through the inevitable challenges. At the risk of being cliche, we truly are seeing everything now as the miracle it always was. There's nothing like almost losing your life to help you appreciate it.

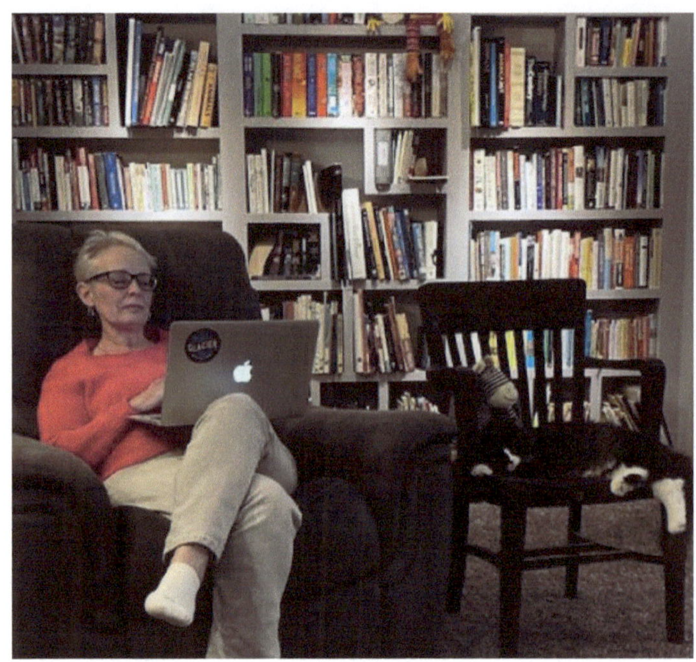

Meet Natalie Mcdonald

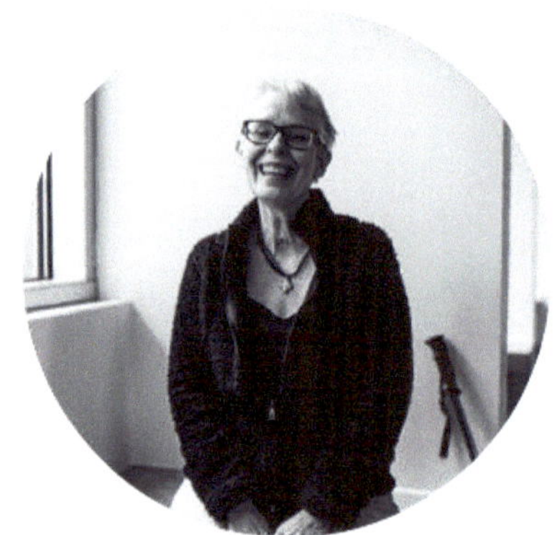

Natalie McDonald lives with her husband Marty outside of Des Moines, Iowa. They have four adult children, Alanna, Ali, Nate, and Evan, and two amazing granddaughters. Natalie suffered a TBI in a car crash in Sept 2014.   She was in level 1 coma for 2 months: she was first in ICU then transferred to another section of the hospital. Before Thanksgiving she was taken to On With Life, a brain injury rehabilitation center in Ankeny, IA.   By mid- January she improved enough to come home and stay. She returns to On With Life regularly for outpatient therapy and to speak at survivor panels. You can read more at Natalie's blog at wordblooms.wordpress.com!

"Let us be grateful to the people who make us happy; they are the charming gardeners who make our souls blossom." *- Marcel Proust*

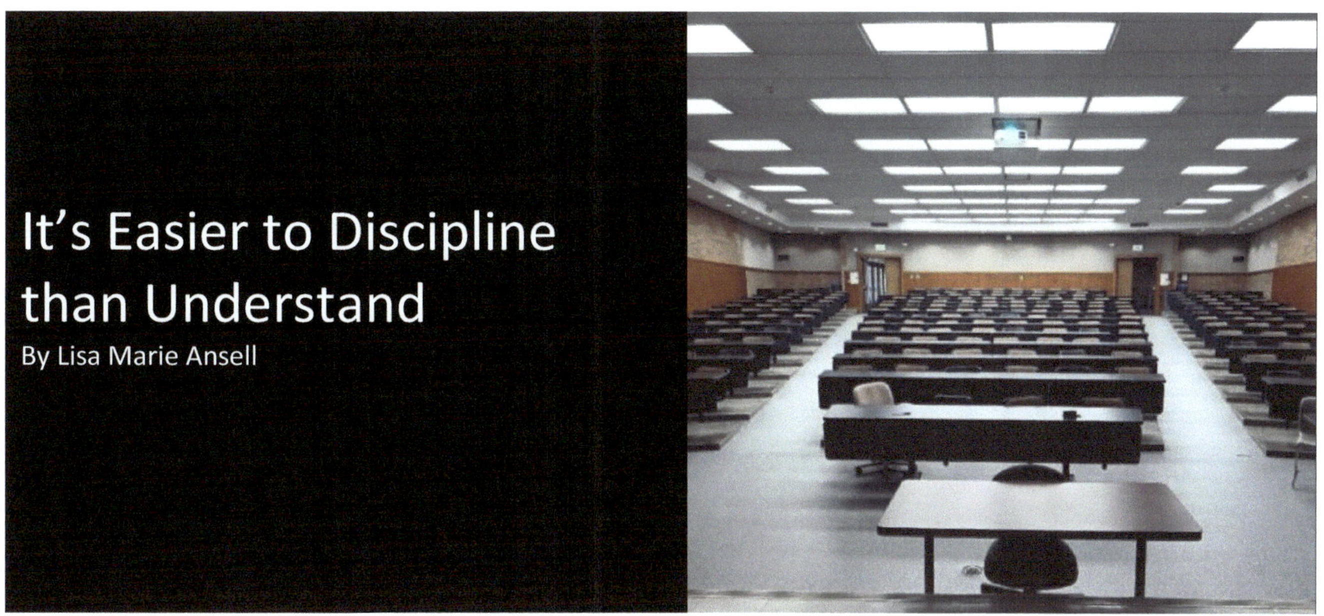

In the spring of 2021, *Hope Magazine* shared my story as a traumatic brain injury survivor. I discussed how education had become part of my rehabilitation and was a big part of my life. For years, I have been trying to overcome my inward feelings of inadequacy for not being "normal" or the person I once was. Misguided, I thought each course I completed or degree I earned would fill that void. After completing three degrees, I found out the last degree I earned was not the appropriate accreditation to pursue my goal of becoming a professor full-time instead of inconsistent adjunct faculty assignments. Halfway through the new degree program, I ran into a huge problem.

I am not sharing this story for myself. I am sharing my story because over sixty-one million Americans live with a disability, with 26% of the sixty-one million Americans living with an invisible disability. People with cognitive issues such as memory and difficulty concentrating or making decisions are 10.8% of people with functional disability types (CDC, 2021). Since 2008, I have worked to overcome my left hemisphere auditory brain injury challenges. I have been blessed to accomplish many things I was told I would not, such as completing degrees without registering my disability with the universities I attended and needing accommodations. Before continuing with my story, let me share some supporting information.

"I am not sharing this story for myself. I am sharing my story because over sixty-one million Americans live with a disability, with 26% of the sixty-one million Americans living with an invisible disability."

Higher education is becoming more accessible and attainable with online degrees, allowing working individuals and people with dreams, hope for the future, and people who would not usually attend

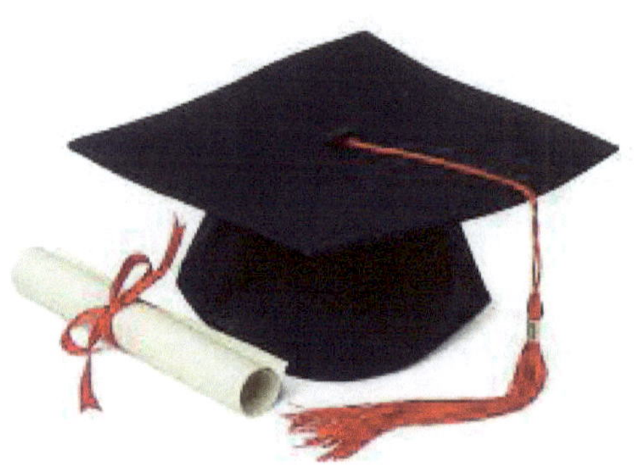

"Many colleges and universities offer accommodations for clear-cut disabilities and allow for extra time for assignment submissions and exams."

higher education courses a platform to achieve their goals. Some students have more obstacles and barriers to overcome than others. Title II of the Americans with Disabilities Act (1990) prohibits universities that receive federal funding, such as financial aid from the United States Department of Education, from discriminating against individuals with disabilities. Students are not required to register their disability with a university to participate if they are accepted into a degree program. One in ten post-secondary students has a disability. Among those with disabilities, 1 in 4 students has an invisible disability.

Many colleges and universities offer accommodations for clear-cut disabilities and allow for extra time for assignment submissions and exams. There are limited accommodations for cognitive processing or visual accommodations, such as transcription services for lectures. Educators are trained to respond when they receive an accommodation notice for a student, which does not identify the disability a student may have or address other accommodations a student may need beyond what the universities offer. Less than half of students with invisible disabilities do not report their disability to the college or university due to perceived repercussions they may face. Exploitation, shame, and unnecessary reprimand and remediation are among the top reasons for non-disclosure, which brings me back to my story.

I am over halfway through a Ph.D. program at a private university that receives funding from the US Department of Education through financial aid assistance, requiring the university to adhere to Title II of the Americans with Disabilities Act (1990), prohibiting discrimination among disabled students (Phillippe et al., 2021).

My biggest fear began to play out nearly ten weeks into a sixteen-week course, halfway through the current program, and three earned degrees prior. I had come so far without my disability being the focus. I was a good student doing what my peers could do without assistance. This overcomer thought I had jumped the hurdle of judgment and insensitivity with people finding out about my disability. Until this course, most of my professors knew of my disability because I CHOSE to share it with them.

During one of the online meetings for the course, there was a guest speaker who had just successfully defended their dissertation. The speaker shared how it still felt weird to be called a doctor. When the time was allowed for questions and comments, I shared congratulations and related to getting used to the doctor title. No harm, no foul, right? Wrong. Those comments started the most humiliating and degrading experience of my life (and there have been quite a few).

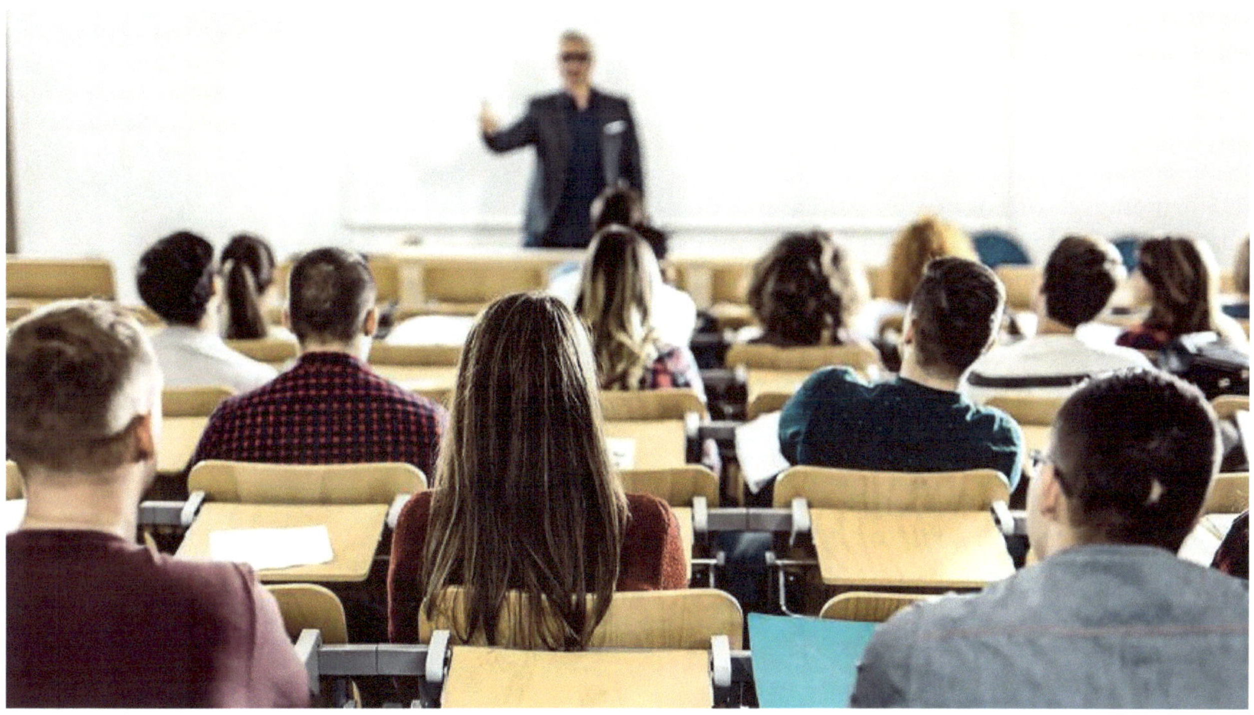

The professors called a meeting with me. One of the professors was not on camera but shared that I "need to be on the same level as your peers." Here begins the chainsaw lashing to my dignity and self-respect. The professor continued by saying that I could not use my doctorate title or experience from my previous doctorate and told me not to mention that I was an adjunct faculty member. By the time this article is printed, if it is, I expect to be a former faculty member as the documentation process for my impending exit has begun. I could not believe what I had just heard. A punch to the gut, the wind knocked out me, trying to process the chopping down I had swiftly experienced. If the professor was going to knock me down to the same level as my peers, they went past my peers and straight to the cow pasture because I felt like I was now among the cow pies on the field. As the other professor asked me to share my feelings with them, I was trying to regulate my emotions to avoid saying anything that would further escalate the situation. Emotion regulation techniques I learned in my rehabilitation process were working overtime. I wanted to tell the professors where the hot place is down south, but instead, I said I did not wish to share my feelings.

The professor would not accept or respect my boundary and again asked me to share my feelings. I took several deep breaths and, at one point, closed my eyes and prayed for the strength to keep my mouth shut. I was again pressured to share my feelings. There was no way I would share my feelings with two people who disrespected me and chopped me down to the exposed roots. Inwardly, I grew angrier with the lack of respect for my boundary. I replied with something close to out of my respect for them as my professors and respect that we are also faculty member colleagues.

I did not wish to share my feelings with them because my feelings were not appropriate to share at the time. Guess what the response was; they wanted me to share my feelings. By this point, I had enough of not being heard and my boundaries not being respected, so I said if they had nothing else for me, I wanted to leave the discussion. I waited for a response and got a disapproving look from the professor who had her camera on while the other did not. I wished them a good day and left the meeting.

After each day of the week-long online meeting session, students were asked to write about what they had learned. On the last day, I submitted a page summary about how through being disrespected, I found a balance between the discussion and working on a level with my peers. Harmless right? Wrong. The professors requested another meeting. I had enough of them the first time. I got in trouble for not sharing my feelings, and now I am getting in trouble for sharing my feelings. The whiplash effect was unbelievable. My faculty advisor held a meeting to officially discuss my "behavioral issues." The advisor spoke about my producing work when group members were not contributing to group projects and how the professors perceived me doing all the work as my not being willing to work with my peers (the projects won awards).

That was not the case at all. I wanted to complete the assignments. Then, she got to the heart of the matter, my disability. The faculty advisor was the messenger of the program director's "requests that you register your disability with ODAS" (Office of Disability Accommodation Support).

As with the discussion with the professors who wanted me to share my feelings, the faculty advisor acknowledged that I did not want to register my disability but requested that I do so again. The level of insult and humiliation was almost unbearable. I am winning awards for my work, maintaining good grades, and earning three degrees without accommodations or "behavioral issues." Now, my brain injury is being thrown in my face. The faculty advisor admitted the situation was a "tragedy," When I told them that I did not deserve this, the faculty member said, "I agree." The result of that meeting escalated into a meeting with the program director, who listened to my perspective, took notes, drew, and colored as I spoke. The program director listened to me for nearly thirty minutes and said, "I believe you. I am so confused because I know you and have not seen this behavior in you." The request to register my disability became the focus of the conversation. At one point, I was asked, "I am concerned something is going on with you medically with your memory from your brain injury because your version of what happened is a lot different than their version of what happened." When I asked what [the professors'] version was, the program director deflected the question, citing that she was not going there and not going to speak for them. So, my question is, how can I have any memory deficits of something when I do not know the other side?

During the meeting with the program director, I was told the doctor title was no big deal, so why did the situation escalate? I was also told I did not take or apply the feedback provided. I was baffled since the project they provided feedback for and was applied to the presentation won an award. I have been labeled with "behavioral issues" for not being able to regulate my emotions when I did a really good job after being disrespected. Finally, I was told my lifestyle might be problematic. What? I do not smoke, drink, do drugs, have not socialized since the pandemic started, and I stay in my apartment doing research, completing assignments, and grading assignments. I make less than 20K a year, and I am poor. Yet, I sacrifice every penny I make to pay tuition without using student loans.

> "I am facing remediation, suspension, and the likelihood of losing my adjunct faculty position because I said no to registering my disability to the university."

I am facing remediation, suspension, and the likelihood of losing my adjunct faculty position because I said no to registering my disability to the university. *Hope Magazine* shares stories of TBI survivors and provides hope and advocacy. My job and continuation in a degree program may not have bright futures, and I am powerless over the university's decision. But I refuse to have my voice silenced by people who would rather discipline and remove than understand and improve. Improve awareness within the curriculum to educate future educators, counselors, employers, and people in positions of power that people with invisible disabilities; people with any disability have talents, dreams, and skills to contribute to society. Disabilities do not discriminate between race, ethnicity, and socioeconomic status. Why does education? Jensen et al. (2021) published an article discussing why it appears textbooks publish next to no information about invisible disabilities and how to work with people with invisible disabilities. Ioerger et al. (2019) authored an article on the willingness of people willing to work with people with disabilities. The issue is not isolated to the United States. As noted by Langørgen (2020) that reluctance and ambivalence exist among educators in Norway regarding their willingness to work with and place students with invisible disabilities. My point is that I am not the only one who has had a terrible experience. Neglect and avoidance are global issues, not just isolated incidents at a university.

Writing and submitting this article will not solve my problems or the global impacts felt by millions of people who live with invisible disabilities. How can we make a difference? How can we change the injustice and discrimination by those in positions of power who would rather discipline than understand? How can we, as people who live with invisible disabilities, move beyond the stigma and barriers that keep us different from others and labeled as "behavioral issues" instead of people trying to understand our perspective without forcing us to register our disabilities or suffer the consequences? The 30K is spent on a degree program I may not be able to finish is hard to swallow, but what I learned will not be wasted. I learned about advocacy, teaching, and working with others. Unfortunately, I also learned and experienced the harm stigma, avoidance, and bias can devastate, humiliate, and degrade. If anyone reading this has any ideas on combatting these issues within the educational platform, please reach out to me.

Everyone has dreams. Opportunities should not be limited to those who have "abilities," for it is the mentality that they are better that makes them more disabled than those of us who are diagnosed with a disability. Multicultural Counseling Competencies need to include training counselors, educators, and employers on ADA Guidelines. Include the disabled population as an individual. Whatever race, ethnicity, culture, or socioeconomic status you are, let's fight back. Everyone has a gift, talent, and contribution to make toward society. Maybe it is our turn to teach the "normies" that we are just as capable of fulfilling our dreams and that if they open their eyes, they can learn something from us too.

Meet Lisa Marie Ansell

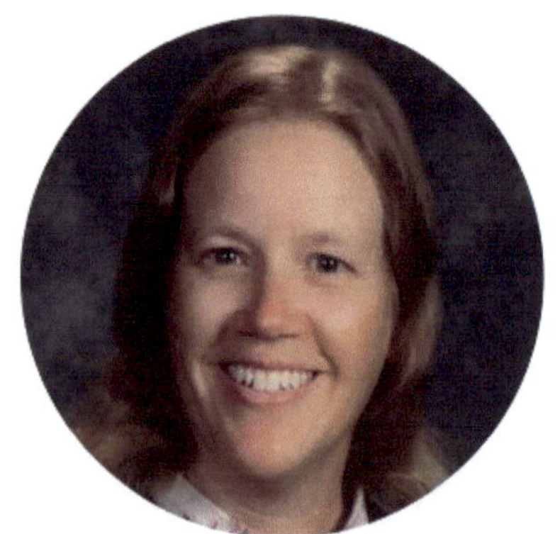

A fourteen year brain injury survivor, Lisa M. Ansell, Ed.D., LPC, NCC, CBIS is a Licensed Professional Counselor, National Certified Counselor, and Certified Brain Injury Specialist. Her hope is that others will be inspired to live their best lives possible after brain injury.

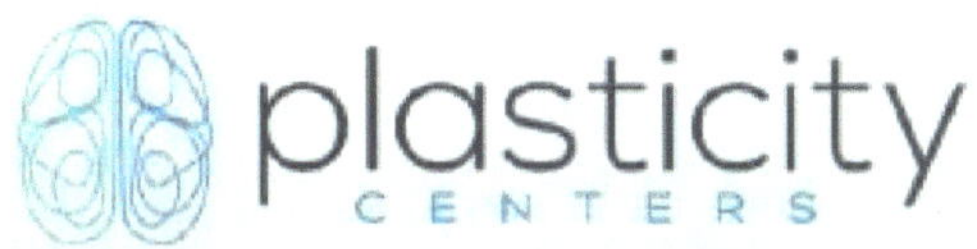

Living With Hope

By Patrick Brigham

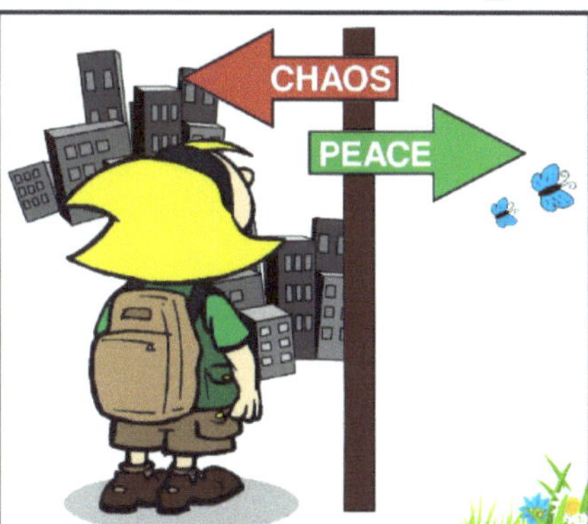

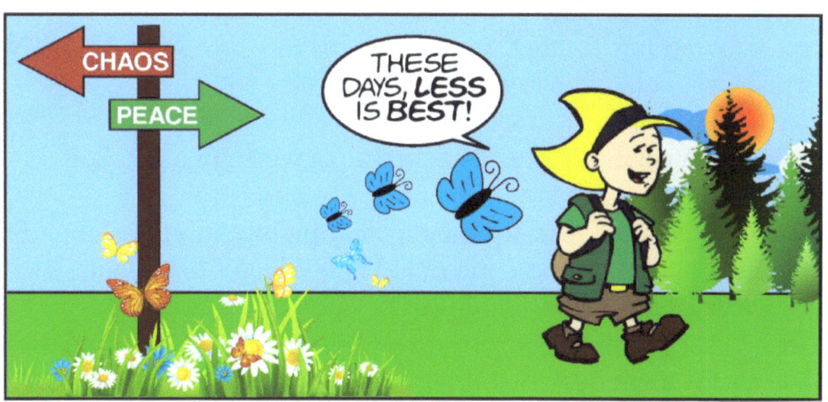

Visualizations & Affirmations

By Isaac Peterson

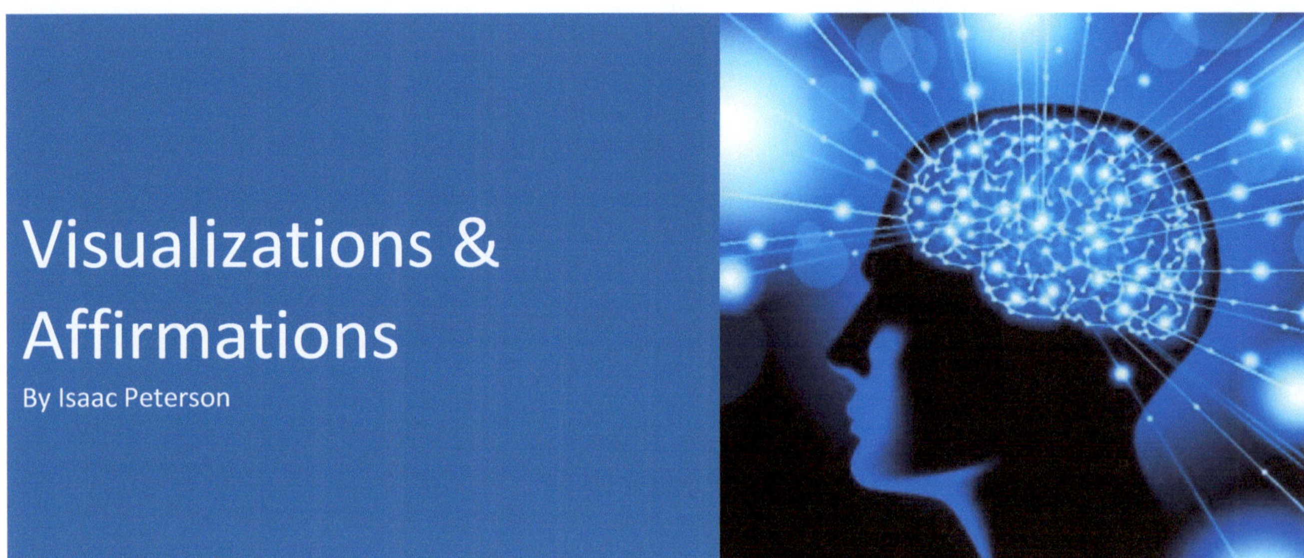

When I was on my month-long hospital stay after a stroke, I began my self-help program while I was still lying flat on my back in bed. I believe what I did there was the real start of my recovery. My body didn't work right, and my brain was still scrambled, but I was still able to do some visualization and I believe that made all the difference.

I remember a few times someone told me something about things I could or couldn't do. I always rejected that. I would say, sometimes out loud, No, it's not going to be like that. I had no doubts I would have more power over my circumstances than they were telling me I would.

What I was doing was not accepting the negative framing of my recovery—I insisted on making my own reality. Since that time, I'm told over and over again how remarkable the rate of my recovery has been. I credit a few things for that, visualization and affirmations, being two big ones.

> "I remember a few times someone told me something about things I could or couldn't do. I always rejected that."

Here's how visualization and affirmations work, in a nutshell.

Visualization is just that; forming a clear picture in your mind of whichever positive result you want in your life and believing completely that you get that result. Visualizing doesn't necessarily mean having a crystal clear image: it can be enough just to be able to feel it, the more strongly the better.

After that, you energize that image through repetition and having no doubts you can attain it.

Here's how it works.

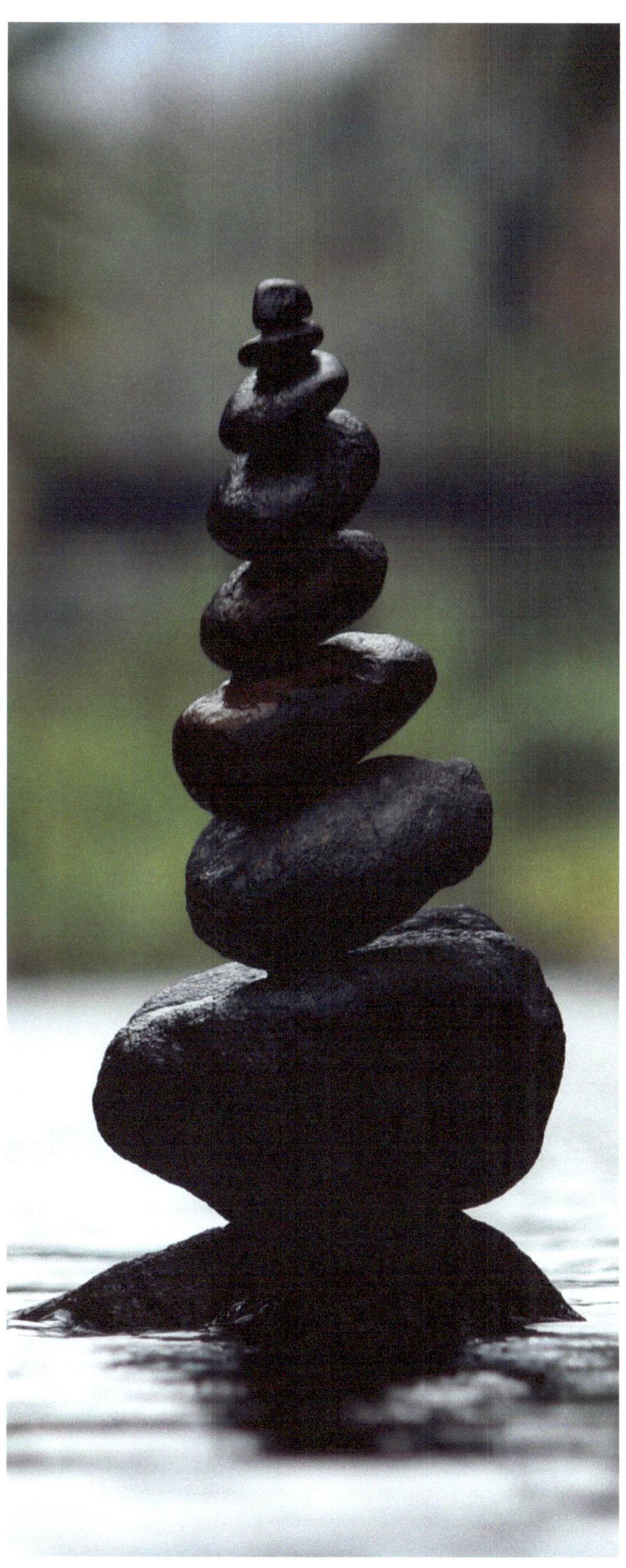

First, get into a relaxed state, sitting, lying down, whatever you do to relax. Relaxing is key: it helps your mind to dig deeper into yourself and concentrate.

When you are comfortable, visualize the change you want to make, and use the most positive wording you can. Figure out what it is you want to see in your life and burn a positive image of it in your mind's eye. To get the best results, don't use negative wording. Don't use words like can't or won't; those words will get in the way of getting you where you want to go.

Avoid telling yourself things like, I want to be…. Say to yourself instead, I already am (what I want to be). I used that approach. I visualized myself in completely good health as if I'd never had a stroke and doing the things I did before. It didn't make me perfectly fine right away; those things take time and I still have a way to go, but I am far ahead of schedule in my recovery as my brain works to restore my mind and body.

Here's another example. If your goal is losing weight, you want to avoid phrasing things like, I won't overeat. It's pretty hard to visualize not overeating without visualizing overeating in some way and defeating the purpose. Instead, try telling yourself things like, I eat a balanced diet every day. I eat sensible portions of healthy food for every meal and I exercise every day. I'm slim and trim and I feel great. Visualize people telling you how great you look. See yourself as already being what you want to become and have no doubts you will get there. Doubt short circuits your efforts.

Our minds (or brains) are there to help us achieve what we visualize. What we tell ourselves will last a lifetime until that message is replaced by a better (or worse) one.

We see examples of this at work all the time. Examples: A child who is told he/she is no good will visualize being no good and grow up believing and behaving that way.

That's kind of how these things work. It comes across like a New Age-y slogan: Think it and be it. But it's not so much about positive thinking, as it is about positive-being.

I find it works best to visualize your goal as something you already have. Have absolute confidence it will come to be. That's what I was doing while I was in the hospital, and it has certainly helped my recovery.

I suggest using varying points of view in your affirmation. Here's an example, using myself as the object:

- First person point of view: I, Isaac, am an excellent writer.
- Second person point of view: Isaac, you are an excellent writer.
- Third person point of view: Boy, that Isaac sure is an excellent writer.

Here's more. Using the example above as a writer, sometimes to make my work more individualized, I visualize part of myself flowing through my fingers, to my keyboard, and into my words. in an effort to give my writing a more personal feel and flow.

I won't become a better writer overnight, but I'm confident I will get there gradually and eventually. Meanwhile, my mind will set up the conditions that will allow me to be a better and better writer.

It could be directing me, behind the scenes, to do things like spend more time developing a concept before I write a single word, figuring out where I want a written piece to go and what the message is, cleaning up typos, tightening my grammar and syntax, and more. It might even lead me to change the way I think about writing, or to eliminate mental blocks that keep me from being as good at my craft as I am able. It may lead me to not try to force my work, but to allow it to happen.

> **"Visualize your goal every day. That helps fix the goal in your mind's eye and gives your mind the focus you need to make it happen."**

Visualize your goal every day. That helps fix the goal in your mind's eye and gives your mind the focus you need to make it happen. Burn the image of what you want firmly in your mind and your mind will work to lead you to the steps you need to get there. I believe this gets to the heart of why so many New Year's resolutions don't work: they lack the necessary degree of commitment.

Visualizing change will work to effect change in yourself, but not to directly affect someone else. It can help you behave in a way that might influence someone else, though.

Let's say there is someone with whom you don't get along at the office, for example. You might visualize the two of you sitting at a table, having a pleasant chat. If it's what you are telling your brain, you may find yourself behaving in ways that will make that person want to talk to you. In other words, you can't change someone else's behavior, but you can change your own to fit pretty much any situation.

As for affirmations, I think it might be helpful to write your positive affirmations down every day for a few days, to keep them in the front of your mind and in your consciousness, until it sinks in and becomes part of your being. This will reinforce your real commitment to that goal. This all may sound like magic, and it kind of is magic, but not in a fictional, storybook kind of way. It's having more power over yourself and your circumstances.

Meet Isaac Peterson

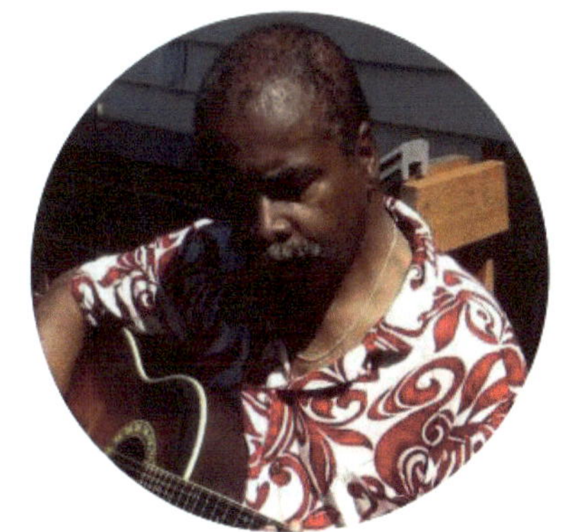

Isaac Peterson grew up on an Air Force base near Cheyenne, Wyoming. After graduating from the University of Wyoming, he embarked on a career as an award-winning investigative journalist and as a semi-professional musician in the Twin Cities, the place he called home on and off for 35 years. He doesn't mind it at all if someone offers to pick up his restaurant tab!

Join Our Facebook Family

What do over 30,000 people from 60 countries and five continents all have in common? They are all members of our vibrant Facebook family at /braininjuryhopenetwork

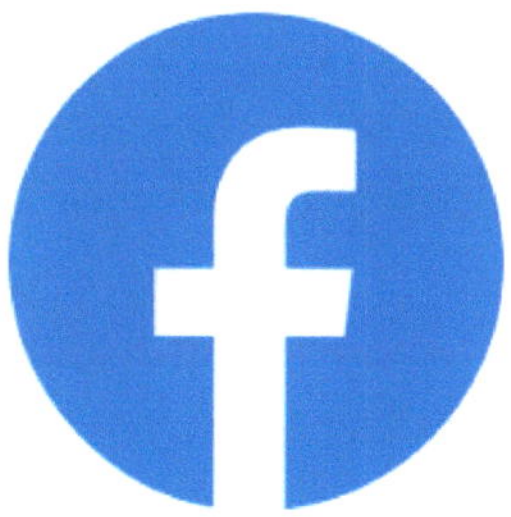

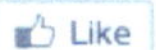

No Last Rites For Me

By Scott Smyth

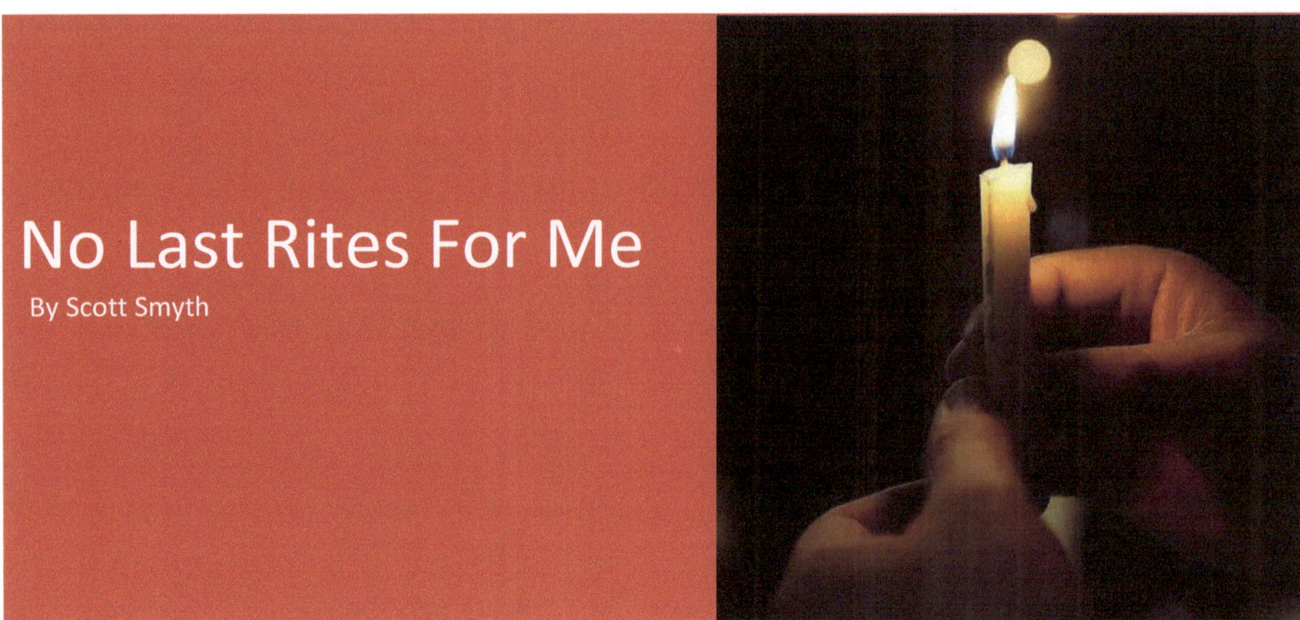

I'm Scott, I'm (gets out calculator) forty-three years old and sustained my brain injury after being assaulted by a group of lads around my age who were under the influence of drinks and drugs. They were later taken to court for attempted manslaughter. Like a lot of us, I was in the wrong place at the wrong time. As for the lads, forgiveness came. in time, and with it, I found peace for myself.

Arriving at home after being assaulted, leaving a trail of bloody handprints along white walls where I lived at the time, I was about to tend to my injured face and sore head when I answered a knock at the door. Following my handprint trail was the chippie owner. I remember thinking "'why does my mouth not work and feel weird?" That was it, I had a seizure and hit the deck. I was about to spend a week in a coma.

My injuries were extensive and included a broken nose, broken jaw, fractured cheekbone, fractured skull, brain bleeding and more. Blue lights on. I have vague recollection of a sea of faces and foggy conversations while under the heavy influence of morphine. Countless get well soon cards from people arrived and I saw more people in a short space of time than ever had around me before, or since. That helped make me realize at the time, I was still thought of, missed or loved.

> "I have vague recollection of a sea of faces and foggy conversations while under the heavy influence of morphine."

Apparently, members of my own family had arranged for my last rites and had plans to turn off the life-sustaining machines. This came to be one of the many things that upset and disturbed me I let it be known how possibly selfish it was as I wasn't brain dead. I seem to have lost the capacity since to bite my tongue. This and other arguments turned my family against me as a brain injury survivor, as well as the changes in my personality, readjustment, the anger, the tears, the acceptance for them that I would no longer be the same person I once was.

I was later diagnosed with depression and PTSD. Those nearest to you don't think it's as bad as it appears. As for memory issues, that's a gripe in itself, not to mention the quantity of pills I was consuming for pain, depression and PTSD - anti this and that – made me feel even worse than what I felt when I took myself off them, against the advice of the doctor who seemed happier to prescribe medication without going into a proper checkup or forward to appropriate professionals outside his practice.

A few weeks later, I was greeted by a letter from my employer stating I'd been terminated for not turning up to work or contacting them. I had an indomitable spirit and the ability to develop a thick skin and probably some attitude with it. When meeting my GP, he said that it was a small concussion he gave me a sick note for two weeks and said not to bother don't bother asking for another one.

There went my trust in this particular GP and many within the medical community. I'm not fault-finding the teams of people that patched me up and send me on my way. They did what they could. I was not given the benefit of a rehab. I was just discharged to family. I was unequipped, under-resourced and had very little follow-up. Suffice to say I had to track down the local brain injury unit for help as this was pretty much before the advent of the internet at home.

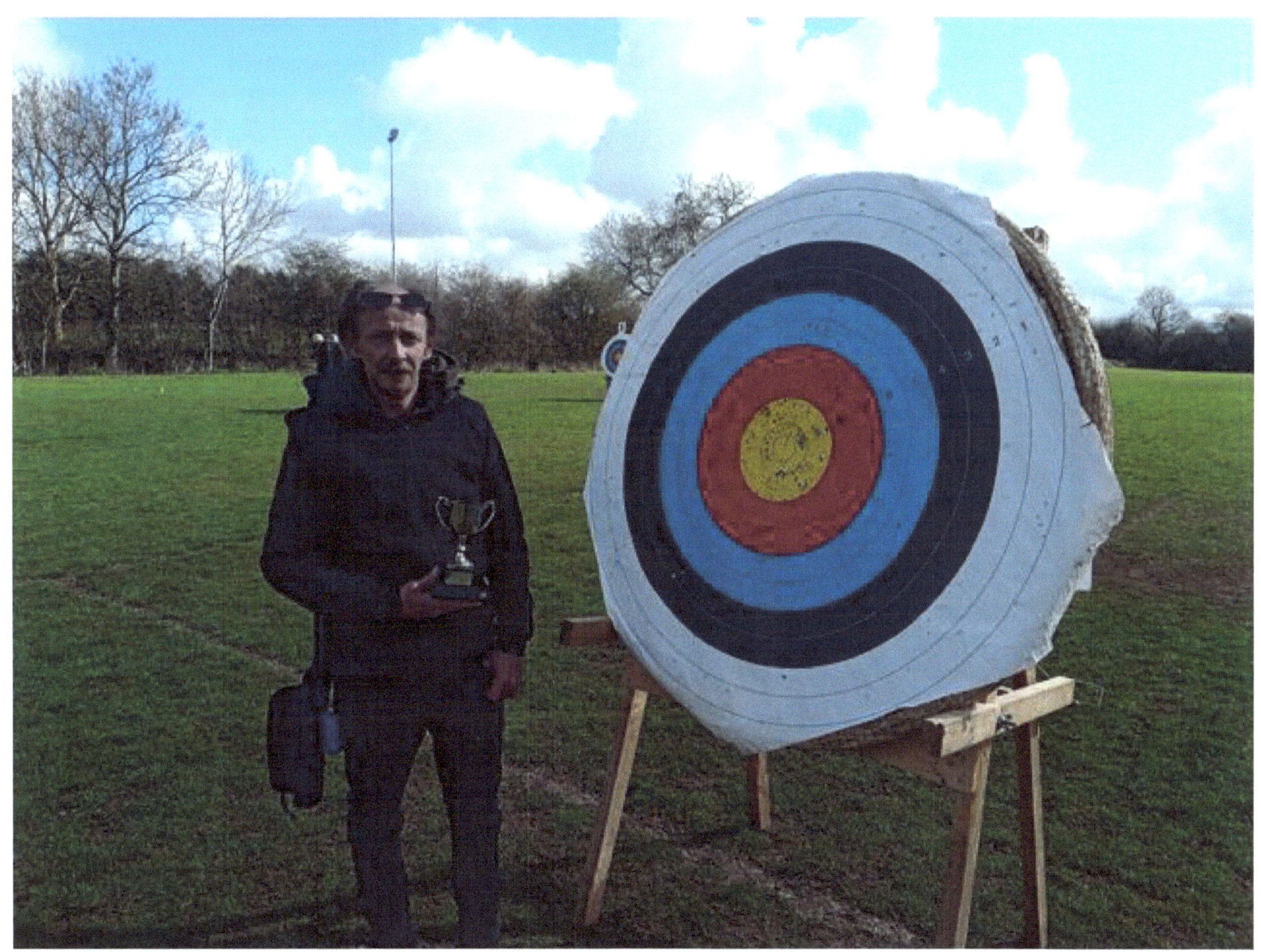

2022 Archery Club Award

During this time, attended some of the local brain injury organizations workshops. I felt strongly coerced by 'friends' to "be a man and get a job" and stop lolling around. Fast forward to 2008 and I was settled with someone with two beautiful kids. Sadly, like a lot of relationships for survivors, it didn't last. She ended up leaving as she couldn't stand to be in that relationship anymore, even for the sake of my kids. My kids still call me grumpy from time to time, but they only know the "new model me." I still never let them see just how hard I struggle on my off days.

I spent time and money going to college and earned some industry-standard qualifications in a few different disciples, including IT and IEEE (Institute of Electrical and Electronic Engineers). These were qualifications that were funded from the result of injury claim. For a career that would span another thirteen years or so, I went on to running my own business for a few years before being taken on by a company I contracted to. Sadly, the recurrences of brain injury issues have a horrible habit of resurfacing and biting us on the backside.

During the same year COVID was coming out, the demons of my brain injury resurfaced. I couldn't do the job anymore, and I was making silly mistakes. Even when I'd written flow charts to aid myself and written my own scripts to make my job easier, it wasn't enough. I was burned out, fatigued and overloaded – even with support from my brilliant ex-employer and other colleagues who sometimes picked up my slack on my bad days

Some days were an absolute nightmare. I was dealing with depression, early starts, not being able to drive due to seizure potentials, medication, as well as dealing with mental processing that was required every day.

> "Sadly, the recurrences of brain injury issues have a horrible habit of resurfacing and biting us on the backside."

Working over twelve hour days working and travelling up to four hours to see my other children each week as any dutiful parent will do, looking back, I wondered how I got through some of those days.

I found myself depressed, with even more worries and yet another failing relationship due to this. This time my ex couldn't cope with my being jobless, being just another person needing to be taken care of with a substantial drop in family income. During the lockdown year or so, I don't think that there's a brain injury survivor who didn't struggle. My hats off to each and every one of you, caregiver, or survivor, that has endured this, with or without support.

For myself, I'd just found myself a new home to live in a month or so before lockdown hit. Was probably the loneliest I have felt in years, with no support and no family visits. There was no travelling - no friends to spend time with. Thankfully, since things opened up, I have undertaken two new hobbies which are active and mental, be it in different ways.

Allotment, a communal garden, helps me just be mindful and at peace, constructing new frames and even a chicken coop as well as a multi-tiered planting bed. I am learning new skills as well as growing food which helps. I have also built a small website to showcase the allotment for being able to apply for grants in the area for funding for tools, equipment, seeds and manure – but no bull! This has now been incorporated into a larger corporate public service site which helps combine my love of technology, and volunteering opportunities which meet my needs.

My time since my injury has not been all easy, but there have been victories along the way. It is my hope that others can feel less alone – knowing that others share the same struggles.

Meet Scott Smyth

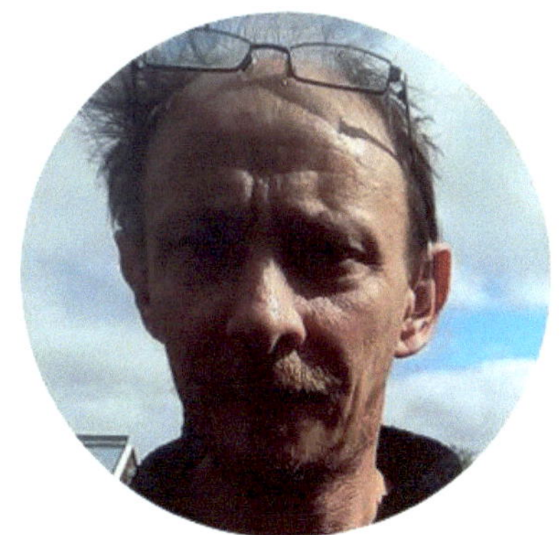

Scott Writes…

"Archery continues to help me in my life. One thing Archery has taught me to concentrate on each small win - each step of the shot. Each step builds up each and the end result will speak for itself. Like brain injury recovery, success comes in small steps. Archery helps my concentration and helps me to better deal with my frustrations in a calm and focused manner. It aids my concentration, It's okay to have off days!"

My Old Friends Depression & Anxiety

By Christina Coates

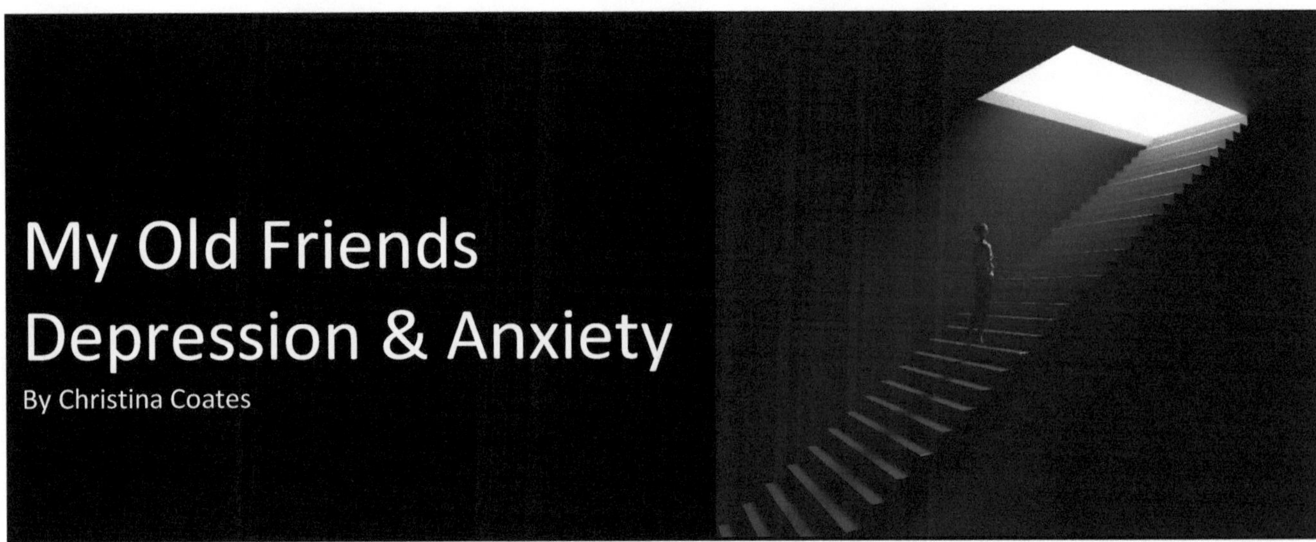

The sheer number of Podcasts that I am subscribed to is mindboggling. One would rightfully wonder where I find the time to listen to each episode. Everything from Fresh Air to Two Disabled Dudes to This Week in Neuroscience. I didn't consider that a Neurology Podcast would remind me that my Rare Disease is always there, even when I drown myself in information and tasks to try to forget about it.

As a child, I remember struggling with what I now know as depression and anxiety. I would cry alone, but I would not have a name or reason for my sobs. I would later learn that exercise, running (in particular), helped me to keep the tears away. I grew to feel that tears were for the weak, and I was anything BUT weak. I remember a day that my spouse complained that he needed to eat because he felt weak. I shot him a glare from across the room and told him to NEVER say that again. Weakness had no place in my life, and I sure as heck was not going to allow my husband to be weak.

> "As a child, I remember struggling with what I now know as depression and anxiety. I would cry alone, but I would not have a name or reason for my sobs."

Leading up to the diagnosis of a Sporadic Cavernous Malformation on my Cerebellum, I had daily migraines. Not weekly, not occasionally, but DAILY. These are not the "migraines" that some people claim to have, which is probably more of a headache. My migraines were very tough. They still are. No matter how much it felt like I wanted to bury myself under blankets and never see light again, I would force myself to get up and go to work. I was that jerk at work who made everyone else look bad because I was always there. One year, I proudly proclaimed to my boss that I "…hadn't used even one sick day…" that year. He was not impressed. Why did I struggle though this? I did it because I didn't want to be weak. I didn't want to give into my depression and anxiety.

When I was diagnosed with the Cavernous Malformation, I was terrified. To be told that you have a lesion in your brain that is right by your brain stem that had evidence of a prior bleed is enough to launch anyone into depression and panic. I went directly into work to warn my boss that I was probably going to have to have brain surgery, which was not at all what my Neurosurgeon and Neurologist told me, but I let the anxiety take me there. In fact, I lived with that little booger for years up in my melon without any problems (aside from the migraines). When he started acting up again in 2020, we decided to have him evicted in 2021. Ah, the joys of needing a highly specialized brain surgery during a worldwide pandemic. That is a story for another time.

After the eviction, I did all my therapies diligently. I was a favorite at Physical Therapy. The surgery affected my balance, so I named myself "The Drunk Baby". I was always of the mind that you should give yourself the degrading nickname before someone else does. That way, you can

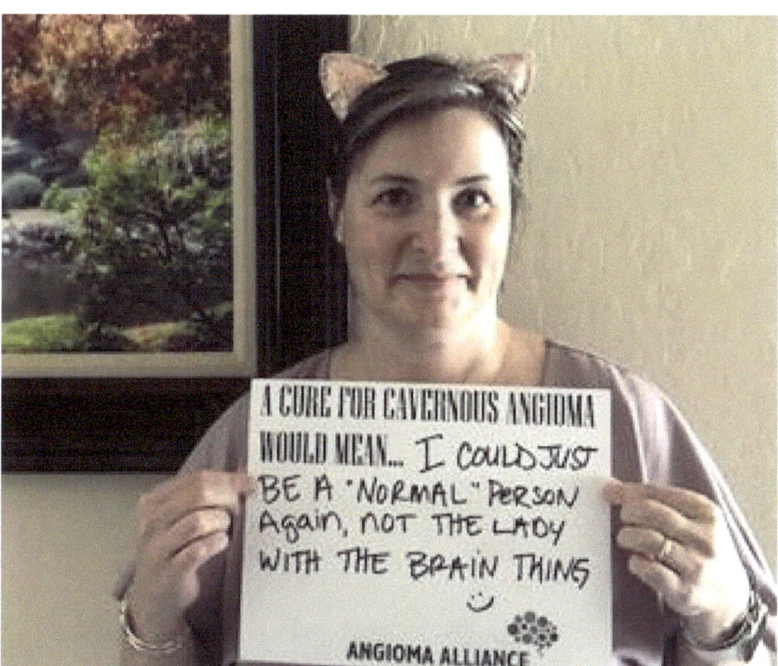

minimize the emotional hurt. When I didn't do an exercise perfectly, I would do it over. The technicians all got to know me well, and when they saw me do something with less than a full fervor, they would look at me, and I would announce that yes, I did plan to do it again.

I eventually graduated from therapy, only to lose the balance and grace that I had learned over all those weeks. I was seeing double. My vision was bouncing. I had spots of numbness in my face and my arms and legs. This is when I was diagnosed with Hypertrophic Olivary Degeneration.

I had known Depression and Anxiety my whole life. They were my constant companion over all the years. I did not know just how dark my mind would take me once I realized that I would never be the same as I was, and that my brain stem was degenerating. I didn't want to live anymore. I made it known that I was willing to live if my husband was alive. After that, I would end it. After all, what would I have to look forward to in life? As far as I was concerned, I couldn't see making anything good out of what was left of my life.

It is unfortunate that we don't seem to have the approach of providing mental help to patients who are thrown into these rare waters. Often, patients are given diagnosis' like HOD over the phone or in a very nonchalant manner. Since our condition is so rare that most neurologists and neurosurgeons don't know anything about it, they treat it as if it is not a big deal. While the patient and family are left to figure out how to navigate this new life.

It has been almost a year since I was diagnosed with the Ultra Rare Hypertrophic Olivary Degeneration. Although I am coping much better now, and I have found value in my continued existence, I still have moments of despair and terror and fear and, yes, even weakness. Yesterday, I was listening to a very technical Neurology podcast (This Week In Neuroscience) that was discussing a paper on Parkinson's and Alzheimer's diseases. It was asked if patients die of these diseases, and the answer kicked me right square in the face. No, these neuro Degenerative diseases don't kill the patient. Usually, it is aspiration of liquid and food into the lungs, or something along those lines. The disease doesn't kill us, it's the stolen brain function that does. And there they were, all at once. My old friends, Depression and Anxiety.

Meet Christina Coates

Christina is the President and Founding Member of the Hypertrophic Olivary Degeneration Association (www.HODAssoc.org). She had a craniotomy in 2021 to remove a Cavernous Malformation on the 4th Ventricle in her brain. Christina has worked in Accounting and Finance throughout her career. Christina works for a heavy equipment company full time, while also running the patient organization. In her free time, Christina enjoys spending time with her husband and daughter, reading, travel, and outdoor activities as her symptoms permit.

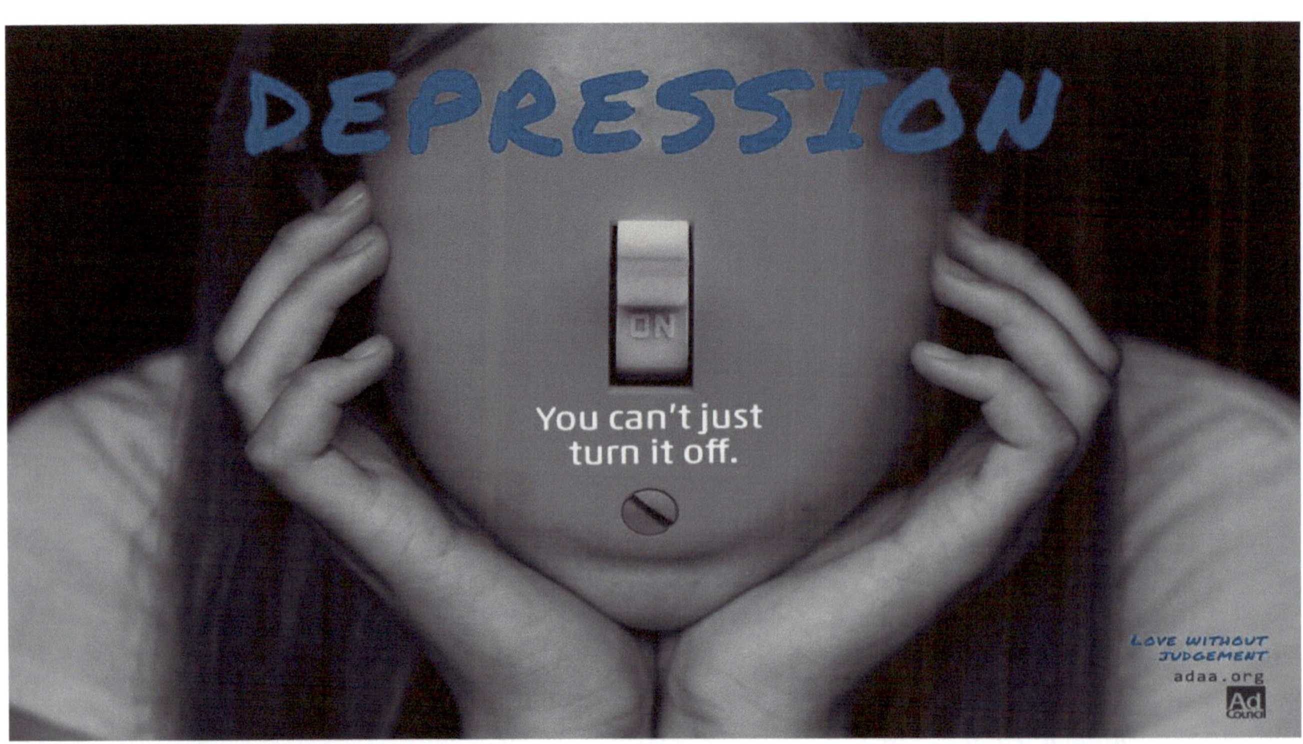

Bumping Into Joy

By David A. Grant

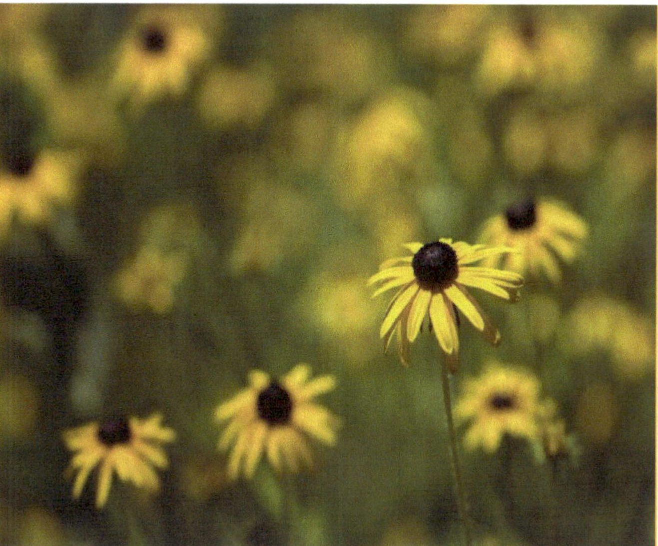

If there was one thing the professionals who treated me after my injury could agree on, it was this: because of my brain injury, I was relegated to living a life with profound challenges. At the one-year anniversary of my traumatic brain injury, a neuropsychologist told me that my recovery was complete and that any gains after a year would be minimal at best. He suggested that I apply for disability, as I would never be able to function at the professional level that I enjoyed prior to my injury.

These were bitter pills to swallow. At that time, my life was a living Hell. Friends and many family members quietly walked out of my life, unable to reconcile "new" David with the person I once was. PTSD was torturous on my good days and downright debilitating on my tough days.

Life at home was tough. Sarah often said that living with me was like living with a newborn, as we both suffered extreme sleep debt, the direct result of bad PTSD nights. There was nothing good about life, and there seemed to be a never-ending wellspring of confusion, pain, and challenges that overwhelmed us both.

> "To be told at this time that life would never get better felt like a death sentence. It is no wonder that suicidal ideation was commonplace."

To be told at this time that life would never get better felt like a death sentence. It is no wonder that suicidal ideation was commonplace. I wanted a way out. Medical professionals were not able to provide it. By this time, a year had already passed, so (clearly) time was not the healer that it was purported to be. I was out of options.

Now that I am in year twelve as a brain injury survivor, I have more clarity than I did back in 2011. I know today that at a year out, I was like a baby learning to crawl. I was very new in my journey and incapable of looking beyond the maelstrom that life had become. I know today that time is indeed a healer of pain, a giver of perspective, and a bringer of joy.

Last month, my wife Sarah and I took a long weekend trip to Vermont. A June Vermont trip has been part of the fabric of our lives for decades. As we do so often, we found ourselves hiking on a boardwalk over a marsh. Birds of all varieties and colors darted about. Sarah spied out a baby snake sunning himself. The wind blew the marsh grass in peaceful waves. We crossed a small stream and watched a few rainbow trout lazily swim by, not caring that we watched them with fascination. In the distance, the sounds of a waterfall created a pastoral audio soundtrack, while the Green Mountains became the literal backdrop of this peaceful scene.

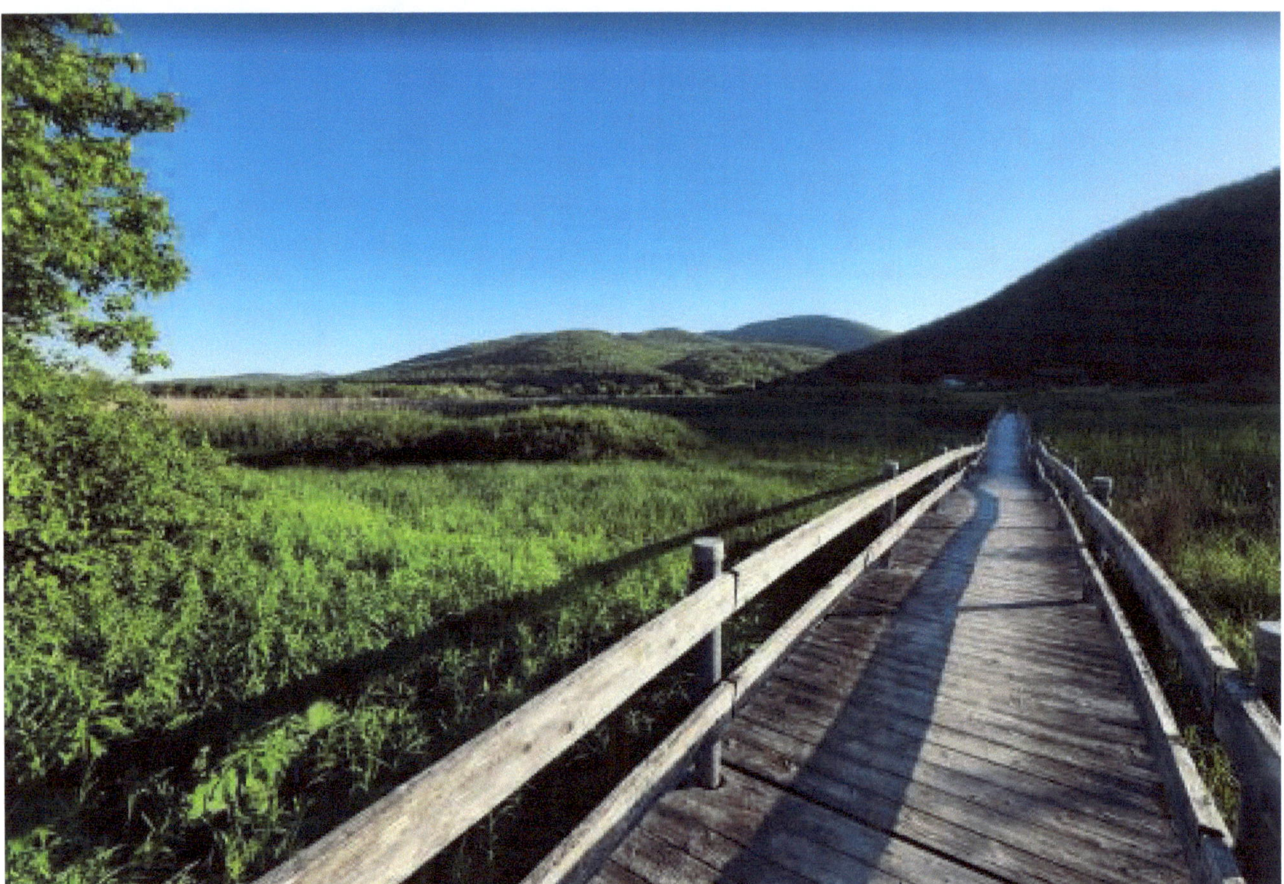

In that moment, one that I will never be able to describe in full detail, I felt an overwhelming joy. It is safe to say that I have never felt as happy as I did right then. I was at complete peace with… well, everything. I had bumped head-on into joy.

This wasn't the first time that joy and I crossed paths. Walking quietly on the boardwalk, my mind drifted to other joy-filled moments... watching the annual return of the hummingbirds to our backyard feeders. Looking out the glass sliding doors at the new deck I constructed this past spring. Walking our local rail trail with Sarah, hoping to see Great Blue Herons in our local rookery. Or, perhaps one of my favorites, our nightly deer safari. We know where to go in town to spot deer. Our success rate of deer sightings is a whopping 90%. Even on those nights that the deer elude us, the very act of heading out on a local safari brings joy.

I can say, without reservation, that these days I am happier and more contented than I have ever been. I am living a life that I never envisioned possible during the early years after my injury. So, you might be wondering how I got from there to here, from the darkest days to some of the brightest days of my existence. There is no way around it, time was (and remains) my friend. For over a decade I've worked tirelessly on my recovery. I accepted that recovery takes time. As time passed, I met a new friend, a friend named hope. I found that when hope is accompanied by joy, miracles happen. I can say this without hesitation, because I am a miracle.

If fate finds you in a tough place in your own life, embrace hope and look for joy. With one hand in the hand of hope, and the other in the hand of joy, they can support you when you stumble. I have found this to be so, and I hope you do too.

Meet David A. Grant

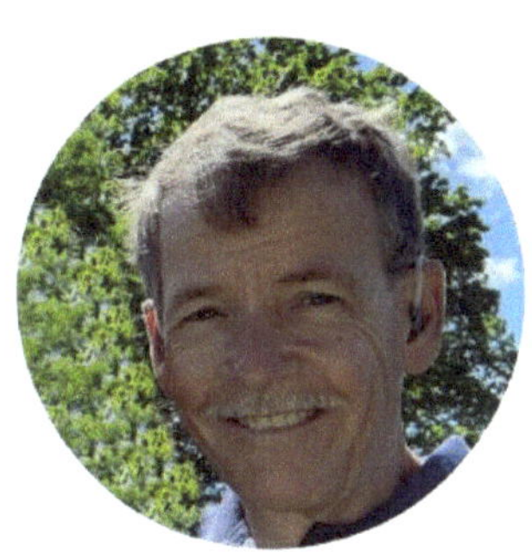

David A. Grant is a freelance writer based out of southern New Hampshire and the publisher of HOPE Magazine. He is the author of "Metamorphosis, Surviving Brain Injury." He is also a contributing author to Chicken Soup for the Soul, Recovering from Traumatic Brain Injuries. David is a BIANH Board Member. David is a regular contributing writer to Brainline.org, a PBS sponsored website.

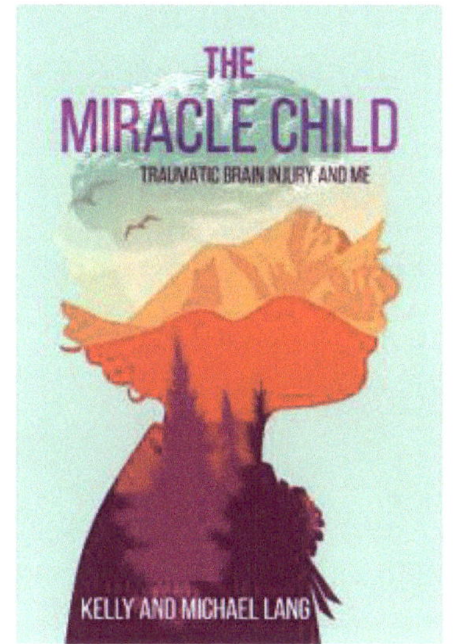

New Book Announcement

Order from Amazon, Barnes and Noble, IndieBound, and more. A portion of the proceeds will be donated to the Loudoun County Volunteer Rescue Squad and the Brain Injury Association of Virginia.

Book Release Date: August 15, 2022

Michael and Kelly Lang's memoir, "The Miracle Child: Traumatic Brain Injury and Me" is a brutally honest and compelling accounting of a tragic car accident that left Olivia, their three-year-old daughter, in a coma with a traumatic brain injury. Readers will be inspired by the Lang's over-riding commitment to family during countless medical challenges that ultimately earned Olivia the nickname, "The Miracle Child."

— *Lee Woodruff, author, "In an Instant", NY Times Best Seller*

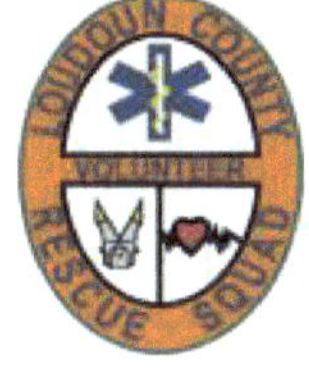

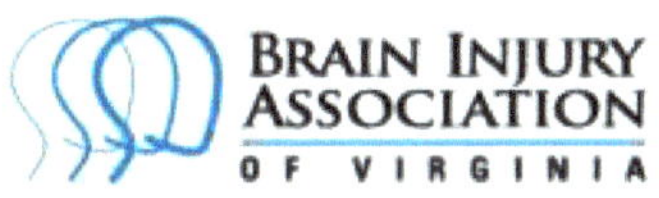

Visit www.themiraclechild.org

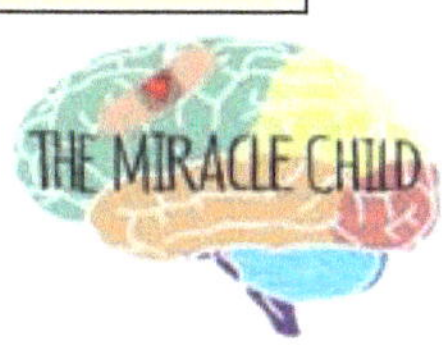

Skydiving Into a New Life

By Mariëtte Loubser

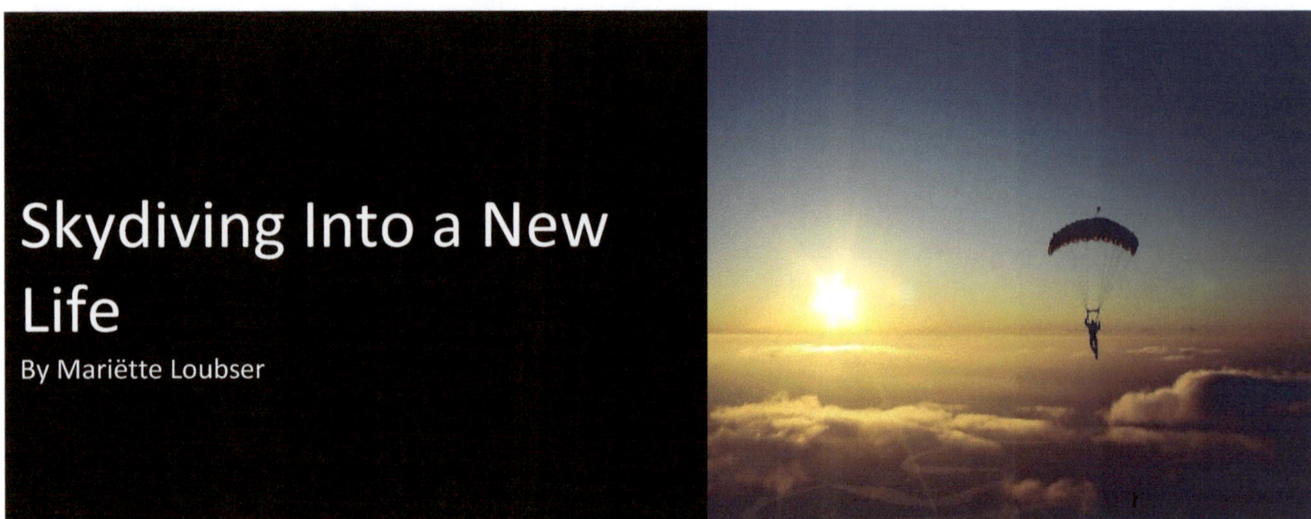

I am Mariëtte Loubser and my story is about miracles. In 2012, I started taking classes toward my master's degree in Inclusive Education. I was a high-school teacher and decided to do a tandem skydive for my twenty-fifth birthday. I found out that I just loved skydiving.

A schoolteacher by week, I was a skydiver on weekends. My first jump was perfect. On my second jump, disaster struck. It was February 23, 2013. Apparently, or so I am told, I started tumbling when I exited the plane. When my parachute opened, the line was blocking my parachute from opening completely. At the time, I was a student skydiver. They kept saying over the radio that I should pull my emergency cord. I was out and just hanging and never pulled my emergency cord. There were buildings next to the landing site. I fell on the rubble.

> "My family and club members waited for the ambulance. After examining me and assisting me, they said that I was too weak to be transported by ambulance."

My family and club members waited for the ambulance. After examining me and assisting me, they said that I was too weak to be transported by ambulance. I was transported by helicopter to Milpark Hospital in Johannesburg, South Africa and arrived at 12:00 PM.

I broke many bones in my back including C1, T4, L4, L5, S2. I broke both my hips - the left one in two places, pelvis, coccyx, and tibia. I broke eight ribs, I tore my lung and sustained a severe traumatic brain injury, as well as a diffused injury. Since I was bleeding internally, I was too weak to be operated on. The head of the trauma unit was trying to stop the bleeding so that they could operate.

At twelve that night he said that I was on the verge of dying and that I could die because I was too weak. However, they needed to operate. I was in the operating room for three hours. They fixed my lung first, then added two plates to my ribs to repair them. After three-and-a-half weeks, I went to Netcare Auckland Park Rehabilitation Centre.

This was to be my home for the next three months. At the rehabilitation hospital, they had to re-teach me things that people take for granted as normal daily activities. My mother was there every day. She worked with me to improve my brain after I was at physio and occupational-speech therapy. My father and brother came to the hospital after work.

I don't remember ever skydiving, nor did I remember much of my teaching and master's program. In the beginning, I was angry at God. Why would he allow this to happen to me? My brain didn't register pain, so I didn't feel any pain in the beginning of my recovery. Later on, I started feeling the pain and I drank many painkillers that didn't actually take the pain away. Besides having pain due to my broken bones, I had a blocked tear gland in my right eye, constant dry eye and eye infections. I had double vision as well. Since my eye moved a lot, I could not get a prism in my glasses to eliminate the double vision.

I am a Type-A person and I started to remember more at the end of 2013. I resumed my master's program at the end of 2013 and began teaching in 2014, only after doing a trial lesson in 2013. Everything was such a struggle. It was like this until I realised that I needed to make the best out of the situation.

An article by Mike Strand in the November 2018 issue of HOPE Magazine puts it into words nicely:

"Stephen Spender has put into words what it takes to succeed with peace and confidence while living with brain injury. I found it all too easy to bring myself down with unrealistic expectations. Trying to be the person I was before my brain injury was the chief unrealistic expectation that I had."

> **"This was to be my home for the next three months. At the rehabilitation hospital, they had to re-teach me things that people take for granted as normal daily activities."**

Things didn't change for me until I adopted a better attitude. It wasn't until I let go of trying to be who I was, that I began trying to be who I could be.

Thus, I decided to make the best of this unfortunate situation. I started joining many TBI groups on Facebook and Pinterest. I read books regarding brain injuries and got tips on how to cope with the situation. I also realized that no matter how much my accident and the after-effects frustrate me, there are people who have it worse.

What has helped me to cope is drinking lots of water to keep my brain hydrated. I read that seaweed helps brain injury. Now, I am drinking kelp tablets. I also read that essential oils help with brain fog and help in having a clear mind. I diffuse different oils to help me. There are days when I am going to have a day that I can't work due to headaches, aphasia or ongoing neuro-fatigue.

On these bad brain days I try to rest, but it is frustrating when I know I have work to do. What has helped me with this is to work ahead so that when I have these days, I don't have to worry about the work I need to do. I also write down everything as I have a poor memory. I put reminders on my phone to help with my memory.

Friends leave after brain injury. You see the true colors of people that say they care, love you and are your friends. My family and God have given me strength to carry on with each day. I finished my master's degree program in 2015. I wanted to give up many times, but my mother and father did not allow me to give up. I graduated in 2016.

I am Mariëtte Loubser from Johannesburg, South Africa and this is my story.

Meet Mariëtte Loubser

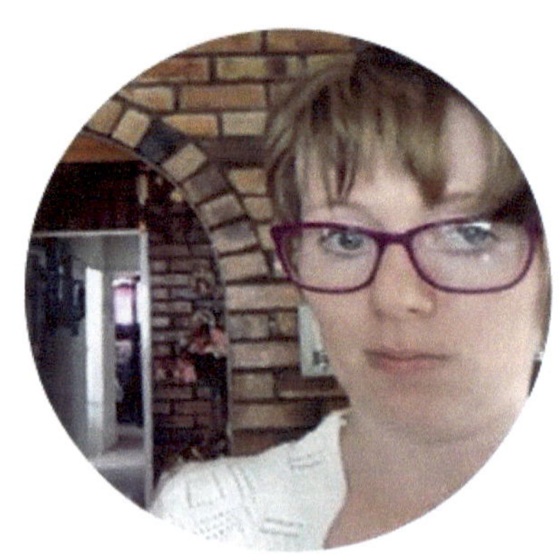

"I am Mariëtte Loubser from Johannesburg South Africa. Currently I am thirty-one years old, but when I had my accident, I was only twenty-five years old. I am currently a high school teacher. I finished my master's degree in 2015. I wanted to give up many times, but my mother and father did not allow me to give up. I graduated in 2016."

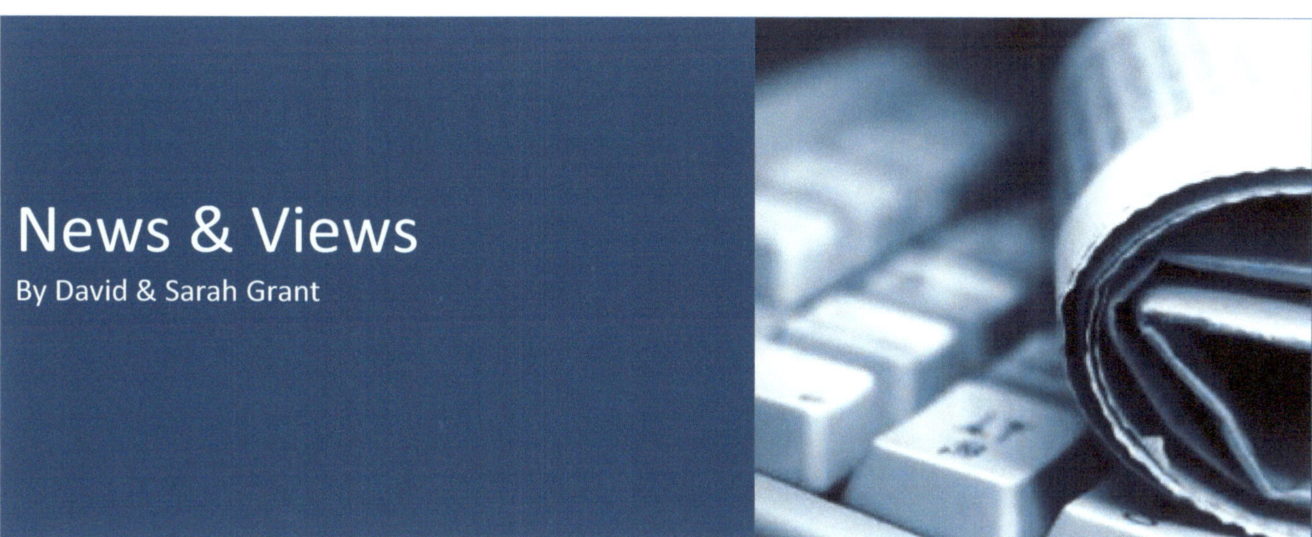

News & Views

By David & Sarah Grant

As we round the corner into full-on summer here in New England, it's difficult not to look forward with enthusiasm. Here in New England, we see the full spectrum of seasons – from cold, snowy winters, to glorious springtime, onward to summer, then the majestic colorful fall season that makes most small New England towns look like post cards.

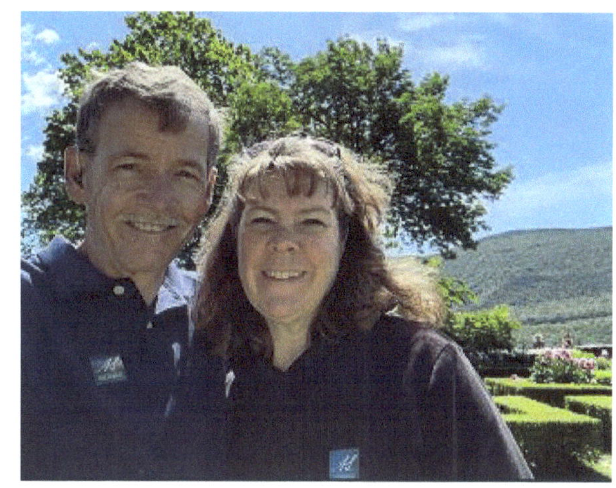

But it is summer that we most favor. Long days and warm nights. Time spent looking for fireflies, backyard cookouts, and the most precious time of all – time spend doing nothing. Summer brings a lot of joy.

As you've just read in this issue of HOPE Magazine, joy can again become part of the fabric of life after brain injury. While many of the pre-injury joys may have changed, new joys can be found.

We are already hard at work on our Fall 2022 issue of HOPE Magazine and have some pretty exciting things in store. We are always looking for new contributing writers. You need not be a professional writer – in fact, we prefer that you aren't. Your story has meaning and can help others to feel less alone. Please consider contributing.

Until next time, be well, and enjoy your summer!

-David & Sarah